MW00509331

The Best Air Fryer Toaster Oven Cookbook

An Unmissable Air Fryer Toaster Oven
Recipe Collection For Your Meals

Eva Morris

TABLE OF CONTENT

© Copyright 2021 - All rights reserved.

The content contained within this book may not be reproduced, duplicated or transmitted without direct written permission from the author or the publisher.

Under no circumstances will any blame or legal responsibility be held against the publisher, or author, for any damages, reparation, or monetary loss due to the information contained within this book. Either directly or indirectly.

Legal Notice:

This book is copyright protected. This book is only for personal use. You cannot amend, distribute, sell, use, quote or paraphrase any part, or the content within this book, without the consent of the author or publisher.

Disclaimer Notice:

Please note the information contained within this document is for educational and entertainment purposes only. All effort has been executed to present accurate, up to date, and reliable, complete information. No warranties of any kind are declared or implied. Readers acknowledge that the author is not engaging in the rendering of legal, financial, medical or professional advice. The content within this book has been derived from various sources. Please consult a licensed professional before attempting any techniques outlined in this book.

By reading this document, the reader agrees that under no circumstances is the author responsible for any losses, direct or indirect, which are incurred as a result of the use of information contained within this document, including, but not limited to, — errors, omissions, or inaccuracies.

Air-Fried Lemon Olive Chicken

Preparation Time: 10 minutes

Cooking Time: 15 minutes

Servings: 4

Ingredients

- 4 Boneless Skinless Chicken Breasts
- 1/2teaspoon organic cumin
- 1teaspoon sea salt (real salt)
- 1/4teaspoon black pepper
- 1/2cup butter, melted
- 1 lemons1/2 juiced, 1/2 thinly sliced
- 1cup chicken bone-broth
- 1can pitted green olives
- 1/2cup red onions, sliced

Directions

1. Liberally season the chicken breasts with sea salt, cumin, and black pepper

2. Preheat your air fryer toast oven to 370 degrees and brush the chicken breasts with the melted butter.

3. Cook in the pan of your air fryer toast oven for about 5 minutes until evenly browned.

4. Add all remaining ingredients and cook at 320 degrees for 10 minutes.

5. Serve hot!

Nutrition:

Calories: 310 kcal

Carbs: 10.2 g

Fat: 9.4 g

Protein: 21.8 g.

Curried Lemon Coconut Chicken

Preparation Time: 5 minutes

Cooking Time: 30 minutes

Servings: 4

Ingredients

- 1 can full-fat coconut milk

- ¼ cup freshly squeezed lemon juice

- 1 tbsp. curry powder

- 1 tsp. turmeric

- ½ tsp. salt

- 1.5 kg chicken - breasts, thighs, or a combo (whatever you have)

- ½-1 tsp. lemon zest

Directions

1. Mix the coconut milk, lemon juice, and spices in a bowl or glass measuring cup.

2. Pour a little bit on the pan of your air fryer toast oven then add in the chicken chunks.

3. Pour in the rest on top of the chicken.

4. Cook at 370 degrees F for 15-20 minutes.

5. Test chicken for doneness by cutting open and observing the center, if you see any pink, cook for 5-10 minutes

6. Use 2 forks to shred the chicken up.

7. Stir in the lemon zest and serve with steamed rice or roasted veggies.

Nutrition:

Calories: 411 kcal,

Carbs: 9.1 g,

Fat: 11.9 g,

Protein: 19.2 g.

Italian Chicken Drumsticks With Garlic & Thyme

Preparation Time: 10 minutes

Cooking Time: 20 minutes

Servings: 4

Ingredients

- 1 tbsp. olive oil

- 1½ red onions, diced

- 1½ teaspoons salt

- 8 chicken drumsticks

- ½ teaspoon pepper

- ¼ teaspoon chili powder

- 2 tablespoons thyme leaves

- Zest of ¼ lemon

- 8 cloves of garlic

- ⅔ cup diced tinned tomatoes

- 2 tbsp. sweet balsamic vinegar

Directions

1. Set your air fryer toast oven to 370 degrees F and add the oil, onions, and ½ teaspoon of salt to the pan of your air fryer toast oven. Cook for 2 minutes until golden.

2. Add the chicken drumsticks and sprinkle with the rest of the salt, pepper, and chili, then add the thyme, garlic cloves, and lemon zest; add in balsamic vinegar and tomatoes and spread the mixture between the drumsticks.

3. Cook for about 20 minutes or until done to desire.

4. Serve the creamy chicken over rice, pasta, or potatoes or with a side of vegetables.

5. Enjoy!

Nutrition:

Calories: 329 kcal

Carbs: 13.3 g

Fat: 0.4 g

Protein: 20.8 g

Collard Wraps With Satay Dipping Sauce

Preparation Time: 10 minutes

Cooking Time: 16 minutes   Servings: 6

Ingredients

- Wraps 4 large collard leaves, stems removed

- 1 medium avocado, sliced

- ½ cucumber, thinly sliced

- 1 cup diced mango

- 6 large strawberries, thinly sliced

- 6 (200g) grilled chicken breasts, diced

- 24 mint leaves

- Dipping Sauce

- 2 tablespoons almond butter

- 2 tablespoons coconut cream

- 1 bird eye chili, finely chopped

- 2 tablespoons unsweetened applesauce

- ¼ cup fresh lime juice

- 1 teaspoon sesame oil

- 1 tablespoon apple cider vinegar

- 1 tablespoon tahini

- 1 clove garlic, crushed

- 1 tablespoon grated fresh ginger

- ⅛ teaspoon of sea salt

Directions

1. For the chicken breasts:

2. Start by setting your air fryer toast oven to 350 degrees F. lightly coat the air fryer's basket toast oven with oil.

3. Season the breasts with salt and pepper and arrange on the prepared basket and fry for 8 minutes on each side.

4. Once done, remove from the air fryer toast oven and set on a platter to cool slightly

then dice them up.

5. For the wraps:

6. Divide the veggies and diced chicken breasts equally among the four large collard leaves; fold bottom edges over the filling. Then, both sides and roll very tightly up to the end of the leaves; secure with toothpicks and cut each in half.

7. Make the sauce:

8. Combine all the sauce ingredients in a blender and blend until very smooth. Divide between bowls and serve with the wraps.

Nutrition:

Calories: 389 kcal, Carbs: 11.7 g,Fat: 38.2 g,Protein: 26 g.

Crisp Chicken W/ Mustard Vinaigrette

Preparation Time: 15 minutes

Cooking Time: 10 minutes

Servings: 1

Ingredients

Salad:

- 250g chicken breast
- 1 cup shaved Brussels sprouts
- 2 cups baby spinach
- 2 cups mixed greens
- 1/2 avocado sliced
- Segments of one orange
- 1 teaspoon raw pumpkin seeds
- 1 teaspoon toasted almonds
- 1 teaspoon hemp seeds
- Dressing:
- 1/2 shallot, chopped

- 1 garlic clove, chopped

- 2 teaspoons balsamic vinegar

- 1 teaspoon extra virgin olive oil

- ½ cup fresh orange juice

- 1 teaspoon Dijon mustard

- 1 teaspoon raw honey

- Fresh ground pepper

Directions

1. In a blender, blend all dressing ingredients until very smooth; set aside.

2. Set your air fryer toast oven to 350 degrees and brush the basket of the air fryer toast oven with oil.

3. Place the chicken breast on the basket and cook for10 minutes, 5 minutes per side.

4. Take out of the air fryer toast oven and transfer to a plate. Let sit for 5 minutes then cut into bite-sized chunks.

5. Combine all salad ingredients in a large bowl; drizzle with dressing and toss to coat

well before serving.

Nutrition:

Calories: 457 kcal,

Carbs: 13.6 g,

Fat: 37 g,

Protein: 31.8 g.

Chicken With Oregano-Orange Chimichurri & Arugula Salad

Preparation Time: 5 minutes

Cooking Time:: 12 minutes

Servings: 4

Ingredients

- 1 teaspoon finely grated orange zest

- 1 teaspoon dried oregano

- 1 small garlic clove, grated

- 2 teaspoon vinegar (red wine, cider, or white wine)

- 1 tablespoon fresh orange juice

- 1/2 cup chopped fresh flat-leaf parsley leaves

- 700g chicken breast, cut into 4 pieces

- Sea salt and pepper

- 1/4 cup and 2 teaspoons extra virgin olive oil

- 4 cups arugula

- 2 bulbs fennel, shaved

- 2 tablespoons whole-grain mustard

Directions

1. Make chimichurri: In a medium bowl, combine orange zest, oregano, and garlic. Mix in vinegar, orange juice, and parsley and then slowly whisk in ¼ cup of olive oil until emulsified. Season with sea salt and pepper.

2. Sprinkle the chicken with salt and pepper and set your air fryer toast oven to 350 degrees F.

3. Brush the chicken steaks with the remaining olive oil and cook for about 6 minutes per side or until evenly browned. Take out from the fryer and let rest for at least 10 minutes.

4. Toss the cooked chicken, greens, and fennel with mustard in a medium bowl; season with salt and pepper.

5. Serve steak with chimichurri and salad. Enjoy!

Nutrition:

Calories: 312 kcal

Carbs: 12.8 g

Fat: 33.6 g

Protein: 29 g

Stir-Fried Chicken With Water Chestnuts

Preparation Time: 10 minutes

Cooking Time: 15 minutes

Servings: 4

Ingredients

- 2 tablespoons sesame oil
- ¼ cup wheat-free tamari
- 4 small chicken breasts, sliced
- 1 small cabbage, chopped
- 3 garlic cloves, chopped
- 1 teaspoon Chinese five-spice powder
- 1 cup dried plums
- 1 cup water chestnuts
- Toasted sesame seeds

Directions

1. Start by preheating your air fryer toast oven at 370 degrees F.

2. Heat sesame oil in your air fryer toast oven's pan set over medium heat; stir in all the ingredients, except sesame seeds, and transfer to the air fryer toast oven.

3. Cook until cabbage and chicken are tender for 15-20 minutes.

4. Serve warm sprinkled with toasted sesame seeds.

5. Enjoy!

Nutrition:

Calories: 404 kcal,

Carbs: 11.3 g,

Fat: 29 g,

Protein: 22 g.

Perfectly Fried Chicken Roast Served With Fruit Compote

Preparation Time: 15 minutes

Cooking Time: 50 minutes

Servings: 12

Ingredients:

- 1 full chicken, dissected
- 2 tablespoons extra virgin olive oil
- 2 tablespoons chopped garlic
- 2 teaspoons sea salt
- 1 teaspoon pepper
- 1 tablespoon chopped fresh thyme
- 1 tablespoon chopped fresh rosemary
- Fruit Compote
- 1 apple, diced

- 1/2 cup red grapes, halved, seeds removed

- 12 dried apricots, sliced

- 16 dried figs, coarsely chopped

- 1/2 cup chopped red onion

- 1/2 cup cider vinegar

- 1/2 cup dry white wine

- 2 teaspoons liquid stevia

- 1/2 teaspoon salt

- 1/2 teaspoon pepper

Directions

1. In a small bowl, stir together thyme, rosemary, garlic, salt, and pepper and rub the mixture over the pork.

2. Light your air fryer toast oven and set it to 320°F, place the chicken on the basket and cook for 10 minutes.

3. Increase the temperature and cook for another 10 minutes, turning the chicken

pieces once. Increase the temperature one more time to 400 degrees F and cook for 5 minutes to get a crispy finish.

4. Make Fruit Compote: In a saucepan, combine all ingredients and cook over medium heat, stirring, for about 25 minutes or until liquid is reduced to a quarter.

5. Once the chicken is cooked, serve hot with a spoon of fruit compote Enjoy!

Nutrition:

Calories: 511 kcal,

Carbs: 15 g,

Fat: 36.8 g,

Protein: 31.5 g.

Lemon Pepper Chicken Legs

Preparation Time: 20 minutes

Cooking Time: 30 minutes

Servings: 2

Ingredients:

- ½ tsp. garlic powder

- 2tsp. baking powder

- Eight chicken legs

- 1tbsp. salted butter, melted

- 1tbsp. lemon-pepper seasoning

Directions:

1. In a small bowl, combine the garlic powder and baking powder, and then use this mixture to coat the chicken legs. Lay the chicken in the basket of your fryer.

2. Cook the chicken legs at 375°F for twenty-five minutes. Halfway through, turn them over and allow them to cook on the other side.

3. When the chicken has turned golden brown, test with a thermometer to ensure it has reached an ideal temperature of 165°F. Remove from the fryer.

4. Mix the melted butter and lemon pepper seasoning, and toss with the chicken legs until the chicken is coated. Serve hot.

Greek Chicken Meatballs

Preparation Time: 10 minutes

Cooking Time: 15 minutes

Servings: 2

Ingredients:

- ½ oz. finely ground pork rinds

- 1lb. ground chicken

- 1 tsp. Greek seasoning

- 1/3 cup feta, crumbled

- 1/3 cup frozen spinach, drained and thawed

Directions:

1. Place all the ingredients in a large bowl, and combine using your hands. Take equal -sized portions of this mixture and roll each into a 2-inch ball. Place the balls in your fryer.

2. Cook the meatballs at 350°F for twelve minutes, in several batches, if necessary.

3. Once they are golden, ensure they have reached an ideal temperature of 165°F and remove from the fryer. Keep each batch warm. Serve with Tzatziki if desired.

Almond-Crusted Chicken

Preparation Time: 20 minutes

Cooking Time: 25 minutes

Servings: 2

Ingredients:

- ¼ cup slivered almonds

- 2x 6-oz. boneless skinless chicken breasts

- 1tbsp. full-fat mayonnaise

- 2tbsp. Dijon mustard

Directions:

1. Pulse the almonds in a food processor until they are finely chopped. Spread the almonds on a plate and set aside.

2. Cut each chicken breast in half lengthwise.

3. Mix the mayonnaise and mustard and then spread evenly on top of the chicken slices.

4. Place the chicken into the chopped almonds plate to coat thoroughly, laying each coated slice into the basket of your fryer.

5. Cook for 25 minutes at 350°F until golden. Test the temperature, making sure the chicken has reached 165°F. Serve hot.

Buffalo Chicken Tenders

Preparation Time: 15 minutes

Cooking Time: 10 minutes

Servings: 2

Ingredients:

- 1egg

  - 1cup mozzarella cheese, shredded

  - ¼ cup buffalo sauce

  - 1cup cooked chicken, shredded

  - ¼ cup feta cheese

Directions:

1. Combine all ingredients (except for the feta). Line the basket of your fryer with a suitably-sized piece of parchment paper. Lay the mixture into the fryer and press it into a circle about half an inch thick. Crumble the feta cheese over it.

2. Cook for eight minutes at 400°F. Turn the fryer off and allow the chicken to rest inside before removing it with care.

3. Cut the mixture into slices and serve hot.

Buffalo Chicken Strips

Preparation Time: 20 minutes

Cooking Time: 30 minutes

Servings: 2

Ingredients:

- ¼ cup hot sauce

- 1lb. boneless skinless chicken tenders

- 1 tsp. garlic powder

- 1 ½ oz. pork rinds, finely ground

- 1 tsp. chili powder

Directions:

1. Toss the hot sauce and chicken tenders together in a bowl, ensuring the chicken is completely coated.

2. In another bowl, combine the garlic powder, ground pork rinds, and chili powder. Use this mixture to coat the tenders, covering them well. Place the chicken into your fryer, taking care not to

layer pieces on top of one another.

3. Cook the chicken at 375°F for twenty minutes until cooked all the way through and golden. Serve warm with your favorite dips and sides.

Chicken & Pepperoni Pizza

Preparation Time: 20 minutes

Cooking Time: 30 minutes

Servings: 2

Ingredients:

- 2cups cooked chicken, cubed

- 20 slices pepperoni

- 1cup sugar-free pizza sauce

- 1cup mozzarella cheese, shredded

- ¼ cup parmesan cheese, grated

Directions:

1. Place the chicken into the base of a four-cup baking dish and add the pepperoni and pizza sauce on top. Mix well to coat the

meat with the sauce thoroughly.

2. Add the parmesan and mozzarella on top of the chicken, then place the baking dish into your fryer.

3. Cook for 15 minutes at 375°F.

4. When everything is bubbling and melted, remove from the fryer. Serve hot.

Italian Chicken Thighs

Preparation Time: 20 minutes

Cooking Time: 35 minutes

Servings: 2

Ingredients:

- 4skin-on bone-in chicken thighs

- 2tbsp. unsalted butter, melted

- 3tsp. Italian herbs

- ½ tsp. Garlic powder

- ¼ tsp. onion powder

Directions:

1. Using a brush, coat the chicken thighs with the melted butter. Combine the herbs with the garlic powder and onion powder, then massage into the chicken thighs. Place the thighs in the fryer.

2. Cook at 380°F for 20 minutes, turning the chicken halfway through to cook on the other side.

3. When the thighs have achieved a golden color, test the temperature with a meat thermometer. Once they have reached 165°F, remove from the fryer, and serve.

Teriyaki Chicken Wings

Preparation Time: 15 minutes

Cooking Time: 30 minutes

Servings: 2

Ingredients:

- ¼ tsp. ground ginger
- 2tsp. minced garlic
- ½ cup sugar-free teriyaki sauce
- 2 lb. chicken wings
- 2 tsp. baking powder

Directions:

1. In a small bowl, combine the ginger, garlic, and teriyaki sauce. Place the chicken wings in a separate, larger bowl and pour the mixture over them. Toss to coat until the chicken is well covered.

2. Refrigerate for at least an hour.

3. Remove the marinated wings from the fridge and add the baking powder, tossing again to coat. Then place the chicken in the

basket of your air fryer.

4. Cook for 25 minutes at 400°F, giving the basket a shake intermittently throughout the cooking time.

5. When the wings are 165°F and golden in color, remove from the fryer, and serve immediately.

Chicken Pizza Crusts

Preparation Time: 15 minutes

Cooking Time: 30 minutes

Servings: 2

Ingredients:

- ½ cup mozzarella, shredded

- ¼ cup parmesan cheese, grated

- 1lb. ground chicken

Directions:

1. In a large bowl, combine all the ingredients and then spread the mixture out, dividing it into four equal-size parts.

2. Cut a sheet of parchment paper into four circles, roughly six inches in diameter, and put some of the chicken mixtures onto the center of each piece, flattening the mix to fill out the ring.

3. Cook either one or two circles at a time at 375°F for 25 minutes. Halfway through, turn the crust over to cook on the other

side. Keep each batch warm.

4. Once all the crusts are cooked, top with cheese and the toppings of your choice. If desired, cook the topped crusts for an additional five minutes.

5. Serve hot, or freeze and save.

Crispy Chicken Thighs

Preparation Time: 20 minutes

Cooking Time: 30 minutes

Servings: 2

Ingredients:

- 1lb. chicken thighs

- Salt and pepper

- 2cups roasted pecans

- 1cup water

- 1 cup almond flour

Directions:

1. Preheat your fryer to 400°F.

2. Season the chicken with salt and pepper, and then set aside.

3. Pulse the roasted pecans in a food processor until a flour-like consistency is achieved.

4. Fill a dish with the water, another with the almond flour, and a third with the pecans.

5. Coat the thighs with the almond flour. Mix the remaining flour with the processed pecans.

6. Dredge the thighs in the water and then press into the almond-pecan mix, ensuring the chicken is completely covered.

7. Cook the chicken in the fryer for twenty-two minutes, with an extra five minutes, added if you would like the chicken a darker-brown color. Check the temperature has reached 165°F before serving.

Strawberry Turkey

Preparation Time: 15 minutes

Cooking Time: 25 minutes

Servings: 2

Ingredients:

- 2lb. turkey breast
- 1tbsp. olive oil
- Salt and pepper
- 1 cup fresh strawberries

Method:

1. Preheat your fryer to 375°F.

2. Massage the turkey breast with olive oil before seasoning with a generous amount of salt and pepper.

3. Cook the turkey in the fryer for fifteen minutes. Flip the turkey and cook for a further fifteen minutes.

4. During these last fifteen minutes, blend the strawberries in a food processor until a smooth consistency has been achieved.

5. Heap the strawberries over the turkey, then cook for a final seven minutes and enjoy.

Chimichurri Turkey

Preparation Time: 20 minutes

Cooking Time: 50 minutes

Servings: 4

Ingredients:

- 1lb. Turkey breast
- ½ cup chimichurri sauce
- ½ cup butter
- ¼ cup parmesan cheese, grated
- ¼ tsp. garlic powder

Directions:

1. Massage the chimichurri sauce into the turkey breast, refrigerate in an airtight container for at least a half-hour.

2. In the meantime, prepare the herbed butter. Mix the butter, parmesan, and garlic powder, using a hand mixer if desired (this will make it extra creamy)

3. Preheat your fryer at 350°F and place a rack inside. Remove the turkey from the refrigerator and allow it to return to room temperature for roughly twenty minutes while the fryer warms.

4. Place the turkey in the fryer and allow it to cool for twenty minutes. Flip and cook on the other side for a further twenty minutes.

5. Take care when removing the turkey from the fryer. Place it on a serving dish and enjoy with the herbed butter.

Betty's Baked Chicken

Preparation Time: 5minutes

Cooking time: 45 minutes

Servings: 6

Ingredients:

- ½ cup butter
- 1tsp. pepper
- 3tbsp. garlic, minced
- 1whole chicken

Directions:

1. Pre-heat your fryer at 350°F.

2. Allow the butter to soften at room temperature, then mix well in a small bowl with the pepper and garlic.

3. Massage the butter into the chicken. Any remaining butter can go inside the chicken.

4. Cook the chicken in the fryer for half an hour. Flip, then cook on the other side for an another thirty minutes.

5. Test the temperature of the chicken by sticking a meat thermometer into the fat of the thigh to make sure it has reached 165°F. Take care when removing the chicken from the fryer. Let sit for ten minutes before you carve it and serve.

Chicken Breasts & Spiced Tomatoes

Preparation Time: 5minutes

Cooking time: 15 minutes

Servings: 4

Ingredients:

- lb. boneless chicken breast
- Salt and pepper
- 1 cup butter
- 1 cup tomatoes, diced
- 1 ½ tsp. paprika
- 1 tsp. pumpkin pie spices

Directions:

1. Preheat your fryer at 375°F.

2. Cut the chicken into relatively thick slices and put them in the fryer. Sprinkle with salt and pepper to taste. Cook for fifteen minutes.

3. In the meantime, melt the butter in a saucepan over medium heat, before adding

the tomatoes, paprika, and pumpkin pie spices. Leave simmering while the chicken finishes cooking.

4. When the chicken is cooked through, place it on a dish and pour the tomato mixture over. Serve hot.

Fennel Chicken

Preparation Time: 5minutes

Cooking time: 15 minutes

Servings: 4

Ingredients:

- 1½ cup coconut milk

- 2tbsp. garam masala

- 1 ½ lb. chicken thighs

- ¾ tbsp. coconut oil, melted

Directions:

1. Combine the coconut oil and garam masala in a bowl. Pour the mixture over the chicken thighs and leave to marinate for a half hour.

2. Pre-heat your fryer at 375°F .

3. Cook the chicken into the fryer for fifteen minutes.

4. Add in the coconut milk, giving it a good stir, then cook for an additional ten minutes.

5. Remove the chicken and place on a serving dish. Make sure to pour all of the coconut "gravy" over it and serve immediately.

Roasted Chicken

Preparation Time: 10minutes

Cooking time: 25 minutes

Servings: 4

Ingredients:

- 6lb. whole chicken

- 1tsp. olive oil

- 1tbsp. minced garlic

- 1white onion, peeled and halved

- 3tbsp. butter

Method:

1. Pre-heat the fryer at 360°F.

2. Massage the chicken with the olive oil and the minced garlic.

3. Place the peeled and halved onion, as well as the butter, inside of the chicken.

4. Cook the chicken in the fryer for seventy-five minutes.

5. Take care when removing the chicken from the fryer, then carve and serve.

Sun-Dried Tomato Crusted Chops

Preparation Time: 15 minutes

Cooking Time: 11 minutes

Serving: 4

Ingredients:

- ½ cup oil-packed sun-dried tomatoes

- ½ cup toasted almonds

- ¼ cup grated Parmesan cheese

- ½ cup olive oil, plus more for brushing the fry basket

- Two tablespoons water

- ½ teaspoon salt

- Freshly ground black pepper, to taste

- Four center-cut boneless pork chops (about 1¼ pounds / 567 g)

Directions:

1. Put the sun-dried tomatoes into a food processor and pulse them until they are coarsely chopped. Add the almonds, Parmesan cheese, olive oil, water, salt, and pepper. Process into a smooth paste. Spread most of the paste (leave a little in reserve) onto both sides of the pork chops and then pierce the meat several times with a needle-style meat tenderizer or a fork. Let the pork chops sit and marinate for at least 1 hour (refrigerate if marinating for longer than 1 hour).

2. Press Start/Cancel. Preheat the air fryer oven to 370ºF (188ºC).

3. Brush more olive oil on the bottom of the fry basket. Transfer the pork chops into the fry basket, spooning a little more of the sun-dried tomato paste onto the pork chops if there are any gaps where the paste may have been rubbed off.

4. Insert the fry basket at mid position. Select Air Fry, Convection, and set time to 10

minutes, turning the chops over halfway through.

5. When the pork chops have finished cooking, transfer them to a serving plate, and serve.

Air Fried Baby Back Ribs

Preparation Time: 5 minutes

Cooking Time: 30 minutes

Serving: 2

Ingredients:

- Two teaspoons red pepper flakes
- ¾ ground ginger
- Three cloves minced garlic
- Salt and ground black pepper, to taste
- Two baby back ribs

Directions:

1. Press Start/Cancel. Preheat the air fryer oven to 350ºF (177ºC).

2. Combine the red pepper flakes, ginger, garlic, salt, and pepper in a bowl, making sure to mix well. Massage the mixture into the baby back ribs. Transfer the ribs to the fry basket.

3. Insert the fry basket at mid position. Select Air Fry, Convection, and set time to 30 minutes.

4. Take care when taking the rubs out of the air fryer oven. Put them on a serving dish and serve.

Bacon-Wrapped Pork With Apple Gravy

Preparation Time: 10 minutes

Cooking Time: 25 minutes

Serving: 4

Ingredients:

- Pork:

- One tablespoon Dijon mustard

- One pork tenderloin

- Three strips bacon

- Apple Gravy:

- Three tablespoons ghee, divided

- One small shallot, chopped

- Two apples

- One tablespoon almond flour

- 1 cup vegetable broth

- ½ teaspoon Dijon mustard

Directions:

1. Press Start/Cancel. Preheat the air fryer oven to 360ºF (182ºC).

2. Spread Dijon mustard all over tenderloin and wrap with strips of bacon.

3. Put into the fry basket and insert the fry basket at mid position. Select Air Fry, Convection, and set time to 12 minutes. Use a meat thermometer to check for doneness.

4. To make a sauce, heat one tablespoons of ghee in a pan and add shallots—Cook for 1 minute.

5. Then add apples, cooking for 4 minutes until softened.

6. Add flour and two tablespoons of ghee to make a roux. Add broth and mustard, stirring well to combine.

7. When the sauce starts to bubble, add 1 cup of sautéed apples, cooking until sauce thickens.

8. Once pork tenderloin is cooked, allow sitting 8 minutes to rest before slicing.

9. Serve topped with apple gravy.

Bacon And Pear Stuffed Pork Chops

Preparation Time: 20 minutes

Cooking Time: 24 minutes

Serving: 3

Ingredients:

- Four slices bacon, chopped

- One tablespoon butter

- ½ cup finely diced onion

- $\frac{1}{3}$ cup chicken stock

- 1½ cups seasoned stuffing cubes

- One egg, beaten

- ½ teaspoon dried thyme

- ½ teaspoon salt

- ⅛ teaspoon freshly ground black pepper

- One pear, finely diced

- $\frac{1}{3}$ cup crumbled blue cheese

- Three boneless center-cut pork chops (2-inch thick)

- Olive oil, for greasing

- Salt and freshly ground black pepper, to taste

Directions:

1. Press Start/Cancel. Preheat the air fryer oven to 400°F (204°C).

2. Put the bacon into the fry basket and insert the fry basket at mid position. Select Air Fry, Convection, and set time to 6 minutes, stirring halfway through the cooking time. Remove the bacon and set it aside on a

paper towel. Pour out the grease from the bottom of the air fryer oven.

3. To make the stuffing, melt the butter in a medium saucepan over medium heat on the stovetop. Add the onion and sauté for a few minutes until it starts to soften. Add the chicken stock and simmer for 1 minute. Remove the pan from the heat and add the stuffing cubes. Stir until the stock has been absorbed. Add the egg, dried thyme, salt, and freshly ground black pepper, and stir until combined. Fold in the diced pear and crumbled blue cheese.

4. Put the pork chops on a cutting board. Using the palm to hold the chop flat and steady, slice into the pork chop's side to make a pocket in the center of the chop. Leave about an inch of chop uncut, and make sure you don't cut through the pork chop. Brush both sides of the pork chops with olive oil and season with salt and freshly ground black pepper. Stuff each pork chop with a third of the stuffing,

packing the filling tightly inside the pocket.

5. Press Start/Cancel. Preheat the air fryer oven to 360ºF (182ºC).

6. Spray or brush the sides of the fry basket with oil. Put the pork chops in the fry basket with the pork chops open, stuffed edge facing the basket's outside edges.

7. Insert the fry basket at mid position. Select Air Fry, Convection, and set time to 18 minutes, turning the pork chops over halfway through cooking. When the chops are done, let them rest for 5 minutes and then transfer to a serving platter.

Spinach And Beef Braciole

Preparation Time: 25 minutes

Cooking Time: 92 minutes

Serving: 4

Ingredients:

- ½ onion, finely chopped

- One teaspoon olive oil

- $\frac{1}{3}$ cup red wine

- 2 cups crushed tomatoes
- One teaspoon Italian seasoning
- ½ teaspoon garlic powder
- ¼ teaspoon crushed red pepper flakes
- Two tablespoons chopped fresh parsley
- 2 top round steaks (about 1½ pounds / 680 g)
- salt and freshly ground black pepper
- 2 cups fresh spinach, chopped
- One clove minced garlic
- ½ cup roasted red peppers, julienned
- ½ cup grated pecorino cheese
- ¼ cup pine nuts, toasted and roughly chopped
- Two tablespoons olive oil

Directions:

1. Press Start/Cancel. Preheat the air fryer oven to 400°F (204°C).

2. Toss the onions and olive oil together in a baking pan or casserole dish. Insert at mid position. Select Air Fry, Convection, and set time to 5 minutes, stirring a couple of times during the cooking process. Add the red wine, crushed tomatoes, Italian seasoning, garlic powder, red pepper flakes, and parsley and stir. Cover the pan tightly with aluminum foil, lower the air fryer oven temperature to 350°F (177°C) and continue to air fry for 15 minutes.

3. While the sauce is simmering, prepare the beef. Using a meat mallet, pound the meat until it is ¼-inch thick. Season both sides of the meat with salt and pepper. Combine the spinach, garlic, red peppers, pecorino cheese, pine nuts, and olive oil in a medium bowl—season with salt and freshly ground black pepper. Disperse the mixture

over the steaks. Starting at one of the short ends, roll the beef around the filling, tucking in the sides as you proceed to ensure the filling is completely enclosed. Secure the beef rolls with toothpicks.

4. Remove the baking pan with the sauce from the air fryer oven and set it aside. Press Start/Cancel. Preheat the air fryer oven to 400ºF (204ºC).

5. Brush or spray the beef rolls with a little olive oil and air fry for 12 minutes, rotating the beef during the cooking process for even browning. When the meat is browned, submerge the rolls into the sauce in the baking pan, cover the pan with foil and return it to the air fryer oven. Reduce the air fryer's temperature to 250ºF (121ºC) and air fry for 60 minutes.

6. Remove the beef rolls from the sauce. Cut each roll into slices and serve, spooning some sauce over the top.

Carne Asada Tacos

Preparation Time: 5 minutes

Cooking Time: 14 minutes

Serving: 4

Ingredients:

- $\frac{1}{3}$ cup olive oil

- 1½ pounds (680 g) flank steak
- Salt and freshly ground black pepper, to taste

- $\frac{1}{3}$ cup freshly squeezed lime juice

- ½ cup chopped fresh cilantro
- Four teaspoons minced garlic
- One teaspoon ground cumin
- One teaspoon chili powder

Directions:

1. Brush the fry basket with olive oil.

2. Put the flank steak in a large mixing bowl—season with salt and pepper.

3. Add the lime juice, cilantro, garlic, cumin, and chili powder and toss to coat the steak.

4. For the best flavor, let the steak marinate in the refrigerator for about 1 hour.

5. Press Start/Cancel. Preheat the air fryer oven to 400°F (204°C)

6. Put the steak in the fry basket. Insert the fry basket at mid position. Select Air Fry, Convection, and set time to 7 minutes. Flip the steak. Air fry for 7 minutes more or until an internal temperature reaches at least 145°F (63°C).

7. Let the steak rest for about 5 minutes and then cut into strips to serve.

Cheddar Bacon Burst With Spinach

Preparation Time: 5 minutes

Cooking Time: 60 minutes

Serving: 8

Ingredients:

- 30 slices bacon
- One tablespoon Chipotle seasoning
- Two teaspoons Italian seasoning
- 2½ cups Cheddar cheese
- 4 cups raw spinach

Directions:

1. Press Start/Cancel. Preheat the air fryer oven to 375ºF (191ºC).

2. Weave the bacon into 15 vertical pieces and 12 horizontal pieces. Cut the extra 3 in half to fill in the rest horizontally.

3. Season the bacon with Chipotle seasoning and Italian seasoning.

4. Add the cheese to the bacon.

5. Add the spinach and press down to compress.

6. Tightly roll up the woven bacon.

7. Line a baking sheet with kitchen foil and add plenty of salt to it.

8. Put the bacon on top of a cooling rack and put that on top of the baking sheet. Insert at a low position.

9. Select Bake, Convection, and set time to 60 minutes.

10. Let cool for 15 minutes before slicing and serve.

Beef And Pork Sausage Meatloaf

Preparation Time: 20 minutes

Cooking Time: 25 minutes

Serving: 4

Ingredients:

- ¾ pound (340 g) ground chuck
- 4 ounces (113 g) ground pork sausage
- 1 cup shallots, finely chopped
- Two eggs, well beaten
- Three tablespoons plain milk
- One tablespoon oyster sauce
- One teaspoon porcini mushrooms
- ½ teaspoon cumin powder
- One teaspoon garlic paste
- One tablespoon fresh parsley
- Salt and crushed red pepper flakes, to taste
- 1 cup crushed saltines

- Cooking spray

Directions:

1. Press Start/Cancel. Preheat the air fryer oven to 360°F (182°C). Spritz a baking dish with cooking spray.

2. Mix all the ingredients in a large bowl, combining everything well.

3. Transfer to the baking dish and insert it in a low position. Select Bake, Convection, and set time to 25 minutes.

4. Serve hot.

Beef & Veggie Spring Rolls

Preparation Time: 5minutes

Cooking Time: 12minutes

Serving: 10

Ingredients

- 2-ounce Asian rice noodles
- tablespoon sesame oil
- 7-ounce ground beef
- small onion, chopped
- garlic cloves, crushed
- cup fresh mixed vegetables
- teaspoon soy sauce
- packet spring roll skins
- tablespoons water
- Olive oil, as required

Directions:

1. Soak the noodles in warm water till soft.

2. Drain and cut into small lengths. In a pan, heat the oil and add the onion and garlic and sauté for about 4-5 minutes.

3. Add beef and cook for about 4-5 minutes.

4. Add vegetables and cook for about 5-7 minutes or till cooked through.

5. Stir in soy sauce and remove from the heat.

6. Immediately, stir in the noodles and keep aside till all the juices have been absorbed.

7. Preheat the Cuisinart air fryer oven to 350 degrees F. and preheat the oven to 350 degrees F also.

8. Place the spring rolls skin onto a smooth surface.

9. Add a line of the filling diagonally across.

10. Fold the top point over the filling and then fold in both sides.

11. On the final point, brush it with water before rolling to seal.

12. Brush the spring rolls with oil.

13. Air Frying. Arrange the rolls in batches in the Cuisinart air fryer oven and Cook for about 8 minutes.

14. Repeat with remaining rolls.

15. Now, place spring rolls onto a baking sheet.

16. Bake for about 6 minutes per side

Air Fryer Roast Beef

Preparation Time: 5minutes

Cooking Time: 45 minutes

Serving: 6

Ingredients:

- Roast beef

- tbsp. olive oil

- Seasonings of choice

Directions:

1. We are preparing the Ingredients. Ensure your air fryer oven is preheated to 160 degrees.

2. Place roast in the bowl and toss with olive oil and desired seasonings.

3. Put seasoned roast into the Cuisinart air fryer oven.

4. Air Frying. Set temperature to 160°F, and set time to 30 minutes, and cook 30 minutes.

5. Turn roast when the timer sounds and cook another 15 minutes.

Nutrition: CALORIES: 267; FAT: 8G; PROTEIN: 2G

Crispy Mongolian Beef

Preparation Time: 5minutes

Cooking Time: 10 minutes

Serving: 6

Ingredients

- Olive oil

- ½ C. almond flour

- 2 pounds beef tenderloin or beef chuck, sliced into strips

Sauce:

- ½ C. chopped green onion

- tsp. Red chili flakes

- tsp. almond flour

- ½ C. brown sugar

- tsp. hoisin sauce

- ½ C. water

- ½ C. rice vinegar

- ½ C. low-sodium soy sauce

- 1tbsp. chopped garlic

- 1tbsp. Finely chopped ginger

- tbsp. olive oil

Directions:

1. They were preparing the Ingredients. Toss strips of beef in almond flour, ensuring they are coated well. Add to the Cuisinart air fryer oven.

2. Air Frying. Set temperature to 300°F, set time to 10 minutes, and cook 10 minutes at 300 degrees.

3. Meanwhile, add all sauce ingredients to the pan and bring to a boil. Mix well.

4. Add beef strips to the sauce and cook 2 minutes.

5. Serve over cauliflower rice!

Nutrition: CALORIES: 290; FAT: 14G; PROTEIN: 22G; SUGAR: 1G

Swedish Meatballs

Preparation Time: 10minutes

Cooking Time: 14 minutes

Serving: 4

Ingredients

For the meatballs

- 1pound 93% lean ground beef

- 1 (1-ounce) packet Lipton Onion Recipe Soup & Dip Mix

- ⅓ cup bread crumbs

- One egg, beaten

- Salt

- Pepper

For the gravy

- 1cup beef broth

- ⅓ cup heavy cream

- 1tablespoons all-purpose flour

Directions:

1. We are preparing the Ingredients. In a large bowl, combine the ground beef, onion soup mix, bread crumbs, egg, and salt and pepper to taste. Mix thoroughly.

2. Using two tablespoons of the meat mixture, create each meatball by rolling the beef mixture around in your hands. They should yield about ten meatballs.

3. Air Frying. Place the meatballs in the Cuisinart air fryer oven. It is okay to stack them—Cook for 14 minutes.

4. While the meatballs cook, prepare the gravy. Heat a saucepan over medium-high heat.

5. Add the beef broth and heavy cream. Stir for 1 to 2 minutes.

6. Add the flour and stir. Cover and allow the sauce to simmer for 3 to 4 minutes, or until thick.

7. Drizzle the gravy over the meatballs and serve.

Nutrition:

CALORIES: 178; FAT: 14G; PROTEIN: 9G; FIBER: 0

Tender Beef With Sour Cream Sauce

Preparation Time: 5minutes

Cooking Time: 12 minutes

Serving: 2

Ingredients

- nine ounces tender beef, chopped

- 1 cup scallions, chopped

- Two cloves garlic smashed

- 3/4 cup sour cream

- 3/4 teaspoon salt

- 1/4 teaspoon black pepper, or to taste

- 1/2 teaspoon dried dill weed

Directions:

1. We are preparing the Ingredients. Add the beef, scallions, and garlic to the baking dish.

2. Air Frying. Cook for about 5 minutes at 390 degrees F.

3. Once the meat is starting to tender, pour in the sour cream. Stir in the salt, black pepper, and dill.

4. Now, cook 7 minutes longer.

Air Fryer Burgers

Preparation Time: 5minutes

Cooking Time: 10 minutes

Serving: 4

Ingredients

- 1 pound lean ground beef

- 1 tsp. Dried parsley

- ½ tsp. Dried oregano

- ½ tsp. Pepper

- ½ tsp. Salt

- ½ tsp. Onion powder

- ½ tsp. garlic powder

- Few drops of liquid smoke

- 1 tsp. Worcestershire sauce

89

Directions:

1. We are preparing the Ingredients. Ensure your air fryer oven is preheated to 350 degrees.

2. Mix all seasonings till combined.

3. Place beef in a bowl and add seasonings. Mix well, but do not over mix.

4. Make four patties from the mixture and use your thumb, making an indent in each patty center.

5. Add patties to air fryer rack/basket.

6. Air Frying. Set temperature to 350°F, set time to 10 minutes, and cook 10 minutes—no need to turn.

Nutrition:

CALORIES: 148; FAT: 5G; PROTEIN: 24G; SUGAR: 1G

Carrot And Beef Cocktail Balls

Preparation Time: 5minutes

Cooking Time: 20 minutes

Serving: 10

Ingredients

- 1 pound ground beef

- Two carrots

- red onion, peeled and chopped

- cloves garlic

- 1/2 teaspoon dried rosemary, crushed

- 1/2 teaspoon dried basil

- teaspoon dried oregano

- **One egg**

- 3/4 cup breadcrumbs

- 1/2 teaspoon salt

- 1/2 teaspoon black pepper,
or to taste

- 1 cup plain flour

Directions:

1. Place ground beef in a large bowl. In a food processor, pulse the carrot, onion, and garlic; transfer the vegetable mixture to a large-sized bowl.

2. Then, add the rosemary, basil, oregano, egg, breadcrumbs, salt, and black pepper.

3. Shape the mixture into even balls; refrigerate for about 30 minutes. Roll the balls into the flour.

4. Air Frying. Then, air-fry the balls at 350 degrees F for about 20 minutes, turning occasionally; work with batches. Serve

with toothpicks.

Dijon Garlic Pork Tenderloin

Preparation Time: 5minutes

Cooking time: 10 minutes

Servings: 6

Ingredients

- 1Cup breadcrumbs

- Pinch of cayenne pepper

- 3crushed garlic cloves

- 2tbsp. ground ginger

- 2tbsp. Dijon mustard

- 2tbsp. raw honey

- 4tbsp. water

- 2tsp. salt

- 1pound pork tenderloin, sliced into 1-inch rounds

Directions:

1. Preparing the Ingredients. With pepper and salt, season all sides of tenderloin.

2. Combine cayenne pepper, garlic, ginger, mustard, honey, and water until smooth.

3. Dip pork rounds into the honey mixture and then into breadcrumbs, ensuring they all get coated well.

4. Place coated pork rounds into your Cuisinart air fryer oven.

5. Air Frying. Set temperature to 400°F, and set time to 10 minutes. Cook 10 minutes at 400 degrees. Flip and then cook an additional 5 minutes until golden in color.

Nutrition:

PER SERVING: CALORIES: 423; FAT: 18G;
PROTEIN:31G; SUGAR:3G

Pork Neck With Salad

Preparation Time: 10minutes

Cooking time: 12 minutes

Servings: 2

Ingredients

For Pork:

- 1tablespoon soy sauce

- 1tablespoon fish sauce

- ½ tablespoon oyster sauce

- ½ pound pork neck

For Salad:

- 1ripe tomato, sliced tickly

- 8-10Thai shallots, sliced

- 1scallion, chopped

- 1bunch fresh basil leaves

- 1bunch fresh cilantro leaves

For Dressing:

- 3tablespoons fish sauce

- 2tablespoons olive oil

- 1teaspoon apple cider vinegar

- 1tablespoon palm sugar

- 2bird eye chili

- 1tablespoon garlic, minced

Directions:

1. Preparing the Ingredients. For pork in a bowl, mix together all ingredients except pork.

2. Add pork neck and coat with marinade evenly. Refrigerate for about 2-3 hours.

3. Preheat the Cuisinart air fryer oven to 340 degrees F.

4. Air Frying. Place the pork neck onto a grill pan. Cook for about 12 minutes.

5. Meanwhile, in a large salad bowl, mix together all salad ingredients.

6. In a bowl, add all dressing ingredients and beat till well combined.

7. Remove pork neck from Air fryer oven and cut into desired slices.

8. Place pork slices over salad.

Chinese Braised Pork Belly

Preparation Time: 5minutes

Cooking time: 20 minutes

Servings: 8

Ingredients

1 lb. Pork Belly, sliced

1 Tbsp. Oyster Sauce

1 Tbsp. Sugar

2 Red Fermented Bean Curds

1 Tbsp. Red Fermented Bean Curd Paste

1 Tbsp. Cooking Wine

1/2 Tbsp. Soy Sauce

1 Tsp. Sesame Oil

1 Cup All Purpose Flour

Directions:

1. Preparing the Ingredients. Preheat the Cuisinart air fryer oven to 390 degrees.

2. In a small bowl, mix all ingredients and rub the pork thoroughly with this mixture

3. Set aside to marinate for at least 30 minutes or preferably overnight for the flavors to permeate the meat

4. Coat each marinated pork belly slice in flour and place in the Cuisinart air fryer oven tray

5. Air Frying. Cook for 15 to 20 minutes until crispy and tender.

Air Fryer Sweet And Sour Pork

Preparation Time: 10minutes

Cooking time: 12 minutes

Servings: 6

Ingredients

- 3tbsp. olive oil

- 1/16 tsp. Chinese Five Spice

- ¼ tsp. pepper

- ½ tsp. sea salt

- 1tsp. pure sesame oil

- 2eggs

- 1C. almond flour

- 2pounds pork, sliced into chunks

- Sweet and Sour Sauce:

- ¼ tsp. sea salt

- ½ tsp. garlic powder

- 1tbsp. low-sodium soy sauce

- ½ C. rice vinegar

- 5tbsp. tomato paste

- 1/8 tsp. water

- ½ C. sweetener of choice

Directions:

1. Preparing the Ingredients. To make the dipping sauce, whisk all sauce ingredients together over medium heat, stirring 5 minutes. Simmer uncovered 5 minutes till thickened.

2. Meanwhile, combine almond flour, five spice, pepper, and salt.

3. In another bowl, mix eggs with sesame oil.

4. Dredge pork in flour mixture and then in egg mixture. Shake any excess off before adding to air fryer rack/basket.

5. Air Frying. Set temperature to 340°F, and set time to 12 minutes.

6. Serve with sweet and sour dipping sauce!

Nutrition:

PER SERVING: CALORIES: 371; FAT: 17G;
PROTEIN:27G; SUGAR:1G

Juicy Pork Ribs Ole

Preparation Time: 10minutes

Cooking time: 25 minutes

Servings: 4

Ingredients

- 1rack of pork ribs

- 1/2 cup low-fat milk

- 1tablespoon envelope taco seasoning mix

- 1can tomato sauce

- 1/2 teaspoon ground black pepper

- 1teaspoon seasoned salt

- 1tablespoon cornstarch

- 1teaspoon canola oil

Directions:

1. Preparing the Ingredients. Place all ingredients in a mixing dish; let them marinate for 1 hour.

2. Air Frying. Cook the marinated ribs approximately 25 minutes at 390 degrees F

3. Work with batches. Enjoy .

Teriyaki Pork Rolls

Preparation Time:10 minutes

Cooking time: 8 minutes

Servings: 6

Ingredients

- 1tsp. almond flour
- 4tbsp. low-sodium soy sauce
- 4tbsp. mirin
- 4tbsp. brown sugar
- Thumb-sized amount of ginger, chopped
- Pork belly slices
- Enoki mushrooms

Directions:

1. Preparing the Ingredients. Mix brown sugar, mirin, soy sauce, almond flour, and ginger together until brown sugar dissolves.

2. Take pork belly slices and wrap around a bundle of mushrooms. Brush each roll with

teriyaki sauce. Chill half an hour.

3. Preheat your Cuisinart air fryer oven to 350 degrees and add marinated pork rolls.

4. Air Frying. Set temperature to 350°F, and set time to 8 minutes.

Nutrition:

PER SERVING: CALORIES: 412; FAT: 9G; PROTEIN:19G; SUGAR:4G

Yummy, Crispy & Spicy Italian Chicken Thighs

Preparation Time: 15 minutes

Cooking Time: 35 minutes   Servings: 4

Ingredients

- 500g chicken thighs

- 1 teaspoon red pepper flakes

- 1 teaspoon sweet paprika

- 1 teaspoon freshly ground black pepper

- 1 teaspoon dried oregano

- 1 teaspoon curry powder

- 1 tablespoon garlic powder

- 1-2 tablespoons coconut oil

Directions

1. Start by preheating your air fryer toast oven to 370 degrees F and preparing the basket of the fryer by lining it with parchment paper.

2. Combine all the spices in a small bowl then set aside.

3. Now arrange the thighs on your prepared basket with the skin side down (remember first to pat the skin dry with kitchen towels).

4. Sprinkle the upper side of the chicken thighs with half the seasoning mix, flip them over and sprinkle the lower side with the remaining seasoning mix.

5. Bake for about 30 minutes until the chicken thighs are cooked through and the skin is crisp.

6. Turn once halfway through.

7. To make the skin crispier, increase the heat to 400 degrees, and bake for 5 more minutes.

Nutrition:

Calories: 281 kcal,

Carbs: 3 g,

Fat: 13 g,

Protein: 36.8 g.

CPSIA information can be obtained
at www.ICGtesting.com
Printed in the USA
LVHW080205150223
739570LV00003B/5